K

The Hidd

To take your sexual life to the ultimate level

By Kathy Lee

Table of Contents

Introduction 5

Chapter 1 - What is Kama Sutra?............................12

The ceremony of lovemaking.....................................15

Aspects of lovemaking – from preparation to climax..19

Food for vigorous sex...25

Chapter 2 - The heavenly scent of a man/woman..31

Seductive Scents 32

Touching and feeling each other 35

Exploring the Erogenous zones..................................40

Pleasuring the Yoni..43

Full Body Intimacy...64

Chapter 3 - The Men's Work 73

Flexing Your Pelvic Muscle 75

Virility and Ejaculation 78

Mastering sexual positions 80

Chapter 4 - Post Coital Positions............................96

The Four Stages of Loving Making 99

Treasure the Experience … and Each Other...............103

Chapter 5 - Couple's/ Partner Yoga 111

Stimulates the endocrine system...............................113

Aids couple's intimacy..115

Chapter 6 - Tantra Yoga 118

Tantra Massage..127

Lingam massage 128

Effects of Tantra Yoga 130

Conclusion 132

Introduction

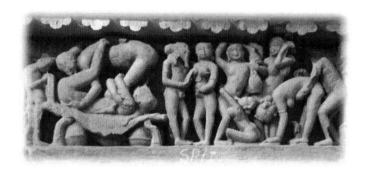

Why should you read this book?

This is a question which arises in everyone's mind because sex seems to be everywhere and needs no description. But if you peep deeper into you mind and ask this question – am I really happy with my sex life – you shall receive a shocking answer – no, I am dissatisfied and dejected with my sex life......... more I get, more the frustration. You are not alone. In fact, a majority of the population feels the same way you do. We are bewildered, confused and shocked by the way our sex lives have stacked up.

We seem to be adrift in this ocean in which everyone is having a fantastic sex life, except us. This book is meant for all those who are lost in this jungle of too much sex but too little enjoyment. It's also for those who are looking for meaning in the act of sex. Love, feelings, togetherness, friendship and bonding are different aspects of sex which will be explored in this book.

This book has excellent illustrations on sex positions described in Kamasutra Yoga and Tantra Yoga. It is meant to be a ready reckoner for readers with plenty of practical advice, both for novice as well as experienced lovers. The book covers different aspects of sex and is not confined only to the physical act of sex. Lovemaking is a beautiful act which combines the physical, mental and philosophical aspects. We have to look at this divine act as a means to achieve total satisfaction. Sex should be instrumental in realizing our goals in life – with complete bliss and happiness.

How is this book different from others?

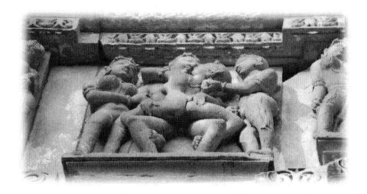

Kamasutra Yoga and Tantra Yoga are subjects which are popular in the Western world. Many books have been written on it. Unfortunately, most of the books on Kamasutra Yoga and Tantra Yoga focus only on the physical aspects of sex. As a result, readers are led to believe that Indian sex is all about sexual positions. Many give up reading such books because some sex positions are quite complicated and can even lead to physical injury. The writers of these books don't seem to know anything about the ancient Indian books on sex.

This book is written from a holistic point of view. Readers of this book will look at sex differently and enjoy sex completely and thoroughly without inhibition.

Another important aspect of sex which must be highlighted is the inability of partners to enjoy sex. Modern day life is hectic leading to many problems – physical and psychological. We tend to focus more on the physical act of sex which can be disastrous. Modern man suffers from impotence, erectile dysfunction, premature ejaculation, low libido and what have you. Women often feel low sexual drive, vaginal dryness, pain during intercourse and so on. This book explores the reasons for such sexual disorders and ways to overcome them. Relationships are essentially built on the framework of sex. Most of the problems faced by couples today have their origin in sex – or the lack of it. Many divorces can be avoided if relationships are nurtured. It's surprising that even in this modern age most of us don't want to look closely and examine ways to enhance our sex lives. This book is a must for people suffering from sexual disorders.

The ancient Indian philosophers were free thinkers. Sex was considered to be central to human existence and was regarded more with respect than as a sin. Sex was considered not only as a physical need but had philosophical and even religious overtones. Sex was considered as a way to reach god. Sex was a blissful union of bodies, an intermingling of souls and an explosion of divine energy. Indian treatises describe the art of sex in detail. Kamasutra Yoga and Tantra Yoga are two important works which are exclusively written to explore the world of sex. These books were written in the days when sex was a genuine desire which needed unabashed fulfillment – not an act which must be performed in secrecy and shame.

The term 'SEX' should normally be associated with uninhibited, explosive, natural, mystic, spectacular, ecstatic, blissful, rapturous and euphoric feeling. Unfortunately, modern day man or woman no longer views SEX in the same way. It's more of an act, which must be performed to achieve orgasm and release – most fail to achieve either. This utter inability to find an outlet to our inner most cravings and desires leads to frustration and despondency. This miserable feeling does not remain confined to sex but spreads across our entire life.

There is more to sex than meets the eye. We live in a world which seemingly is free of taboos regarding physical union between man and woman, man and man, woman and woman. The truth cannot be further from it. Ironically, sex is still considered to be obscene and shameful – to be conducted in darkness and in secret. Some sexual unions are unlawful and confined to the closet. Popular religions prohibit sex unless it's meant to bring children into the world. We are made to feel guilty about our feeling towards sex. There are indeed many obstacles to free sex.

There is another world beyond the forbidden and taboo – mindless and casual sex. You are made to feel that sex is something which you must perform mindlessly – in the backseat of a car, in the open (when no one is looking), in dark alleys and staircases. There is a total disregard of feelings and togetherness. There seems to be no association between sex and love. If everyone was happy with this kind of mindless sex, it would have been great but the fact is otherwise. People are dissatisfied and unhappy with their sex lives because of the casual and careless attitude which leaves us frustrated. This book on Kamasutra Yoga and Tantra Yoga will dispel commonly held beliefs and myths about sex.

This book is a must read for everyone living in the Western world. The irony is that we claim to know everything about sex after a few tumbles in bed or in the backseat of cars. The fact is that we know very little about enhancing sexual pleasure. This book will reveal the secrets of sex – in totally raw and also most subtle form.

Chapter 1 - What is Kama Sutra?

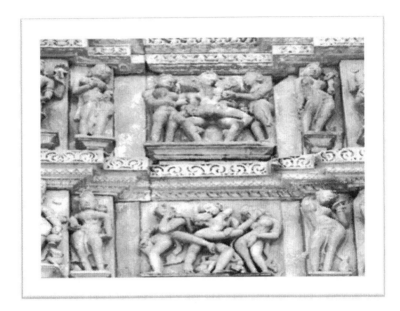

Kama in Hindu religion means desire and Kama Sutra means treatise on desire. This ebook consists of all things related to sex, passion and desire. Most of all it's a practical guide to achieve complete sexual satisfaction. Kamasutra was written by Vatsyayana somewhere between first and sixth century AD. The original 'book of love'

seems to have undergone changes subsequently with more additions and commentaries. As a result, we are now witness to an astounding book on the art of lovemaking which encompasses the entire gamut of sex with all the subtle flavors and intoxicating aroma floating in the rarefied air of erotic mysticism.

Before we dive deep into the mysteries of love and lovemaking, we have to understand the context in which Kamasutra has been written. As we all know, Kamasutra is a Hindu book which takes into consideration various aspects of Hindu life. Sex was considered a part of life when Kamasutra was written. You will therefore discover that Vatsyayana did not shy away from discussing the intricacies of lovemaking. In fact Kamasutra is a free and frank discourse on the desires of the flesh without any inhibitions.

Kama or desire is one of the four goals of Hindu life. Combined   - Dharma, Artha, Kama and moksha are the four goals which human beings should strive for. Dharma is the foremost goal which means righteousness. Without dharma you cannot lead a fruitful life. Artha means the pursuit of wealth. It's believed that a man or woman cannot enjoy life without processing wealth. An empty stomach is a huge obstacle in leading a good life. Kama means pleasure or sexual desire. Your desires can be fulfilled only if you have wealth and don't have to spend all your time working. Lastly, Moksha means escape from the cycle of life and death. Moksha is the ultimate goal of every human being. It has been argued that no man can gain Moksha unless he or she has fulfilled all their earthly desires. A dying person who still desires sex will be born in the animal kingdom to enjoy sex. Therefore, the desire for sex and the fire of passion must fully subside if you want liberation from the cycle of life and death. It's from this viewpoint that Kamasutra has been written. There will be many places in this ebook which you will refuse to accept, especially the sexual positions. You must have an open mind and explore them dispassionately if you want to truly benefit from this book.

The ceremony of lovemaking

Vatsyayana, the author of Kama Sutra clearly states that sexual positions are not as important as the ceremonies surrounding it. In short, the mood is much more important than the sex act itself. One of the main reasons why couples fail to enjoy sex is because sex is considered as something to get over with quickly. As a result neither partner is satisfied. The mood can set desires aflame and the fire will last much longer than the actual act of sex. The lingering, soothing and, satiated feeling can only be created if you consciously work on it. Kama Sutra emphasizes the critical role of ceremony which transforms ordinary sex into a sublime art.

Though sex must be spontaneous and natural, you should try to deliberately build the tempo leading to an explosive climax. The weekend is a great time to have sex. Generally we are very busy throughout the week. Meeting your partner may be possible but where is the guarantee that both of you will be mentally in the right frame of mind for sex? But imagine you plan to have sex over the weekend – the anticipation and expectancy will keep both of you in a heightened state of awareness. There will be a hum of eroticism which you can hear in your mind. Imagine how you will feel and respond to various stimuli during the entire week while anticipating a weekend full of sex and more sex. Titillating for sure.

The weekend retreat

Most of us believe that orgasm is the ultimate goal of sex. This orgasm centric approach to sex means we behave like a pair of fighters in a boxing ring. We start bonking as soon as the whistle rings and stop when we are completely exhausted. If this is the meaning of sex, you can be sure that you will soon get bored with it. This is what actually happens to couples who have been together for some time. Once we get bored (which is inevitable), we start looking for other partners, in the mistaken belief that sex with the new partner would be different. This is an obvious outcome when you don't look at sex as wholesome fun but only an exercise to achieve orgasm. You might as well masturbate and reach an orgasm than spend your precious time looking for a suitable partner.

When you plan for extended sex over the weekend, you will naturally build up the tempo during the week. You can steal small moments to touch each other suggestively, hug and hold each other while kissing fleetingly. You will feel the sexual energy rise inside, releasing hormones. Do not give in to temptation and go for a quickie. Let the feeling simmer inside.

Meanwhile, you must make sure that your bordello is tastefully decorated for sex. You must have the right bed sheets and pillows of different sizes (for accommodating different sexual poses). Remember that your mood depends on the surroundings. Of course you will not be confined to the bedroom. If it's cold outside, you would like to make love in front of the fireplace. During warn sunny days of summer, lovemaking in the open can be a divine experience.

The weekend is going to be long and sex will likely be spread over. You must plan for a quick bite in between bouts of lovemaking. Vatsyayana recommends having fruits and light refreshments during sex. You must avoid eating heavy stuff like red meat because it makes you sluggish and sleepy. There are some other factors which enhance lovemaking. Music can elevate sex. Music should be soothing and soft. You must avoid loud music which distracts from lovemaking. Instrumental music played in the background can be helpful in timing your strokes while your penis is inside the vagina of your lover – starting with slow and long strokes and ending with short quick thrusts.

Music is not restricted to thrusting and stroking alone. Music can alter your mood and make you relax. Listen to music and let the negative emotions, which have built up over the week, dissolve and melt away. Rhythmic music also slows your heart rate and breathing. You can have better control over ejaculation when you control your breath.

Kama Sutra recommends light to moderate drinking during your prolonged lovemaking session. Heavy drinking should be avoided since it may lead to insufficient erection and arousal for men. You may not be able to enjoy sex at the fullest if any of you drink too much alcohol.

Aspects of lovemaking – from preparation to climax

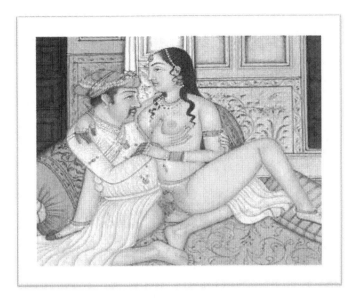

Weekend sex (or prolonged sex sessions) must always begin with seduction and playful romance. Skin is the most primordial sense organ. Touch excites and prepares you for sex. It provides a heightened sense of pleasure and anticipation for things to come. Weekend sex just means extended period of lovemaking, not necessarily restricted to weekend. You may decide to have prolonged session of sex during a holiday, in the outdoors. Vatsyayana suggest that sex should be spontaneous and impulsive, though the planning is deliberate and detailed.

Making love in the open and under the stars is extremely erotic and satisfying. The blue sky above can also give you a feeling of eternity and extreme sexual bliss. In the days of Kama Sutra, people went out for picnics in horseback and camped outdoors. Couples found secluded and open places where they made love and returned to the campsite. Group sex was common during Kama Sutra days. Sex was a divine experience and there were no taboos as long as both men and women enjoyed sex without inhibition.

According to Vatsyayana, all your five senses must be explored to provide complete sexual satisfaction. These five senses are taste, smell, touch, hearing and sight. We appreciate this world through these five sense organs – tongue, nose, skin, ears and eyes. As against this, what do you actually see people doing? They isolate sex act from the experience of the senses – the focus is on sex and nothing else. The result is obviously a disaster. So, what is meant by involving the five senses?

The eye is the first gateway to experience. Our vision usually provides the foundation to all our experiences. Vatsyayana emphasizes the need for visual appeal to derive maximum pleasure from sex. Kama Sutra describes the ambiance and setting in great detail. The first and most used location for sex is the bedroom. Sex is a natural outcome of togetherness and the bedroom provides this in ample measure.

In the days of Vatsyayana, there was no electricity. The night was brought alive with candles and lanterns. People with means had their bedroom decorated with bright colored flowers. The floor was covered with multi-hued designs made out of crushed flowers which gave wonderful and intoxicating smell. The candles were put in places which enhanced shadows and evoked sensuality. The play of light and shadow created a mystical atmosphere which was perfect for extended lovemaking.

We are lucky to be living in this tech driven world. We can create any visual theme right inside our bedroom. A little bit of imagination can do wonders to your bedroom as well as your libido. You must use blue to enhance the feeling of complete relaxation. Red color shows energy and vitality. Use colors of the bedroom walls imaginatively. A splash of red here and a serene blue elsewhere will exude passion, togetherness, love, affection and adoration. The colors will give an impetus to your desires and provoke you to experiment with lovemaking. Every occasion must be unique and drive you to new peaks of sexual pleasure.

Your place of making love must not be too warm or too cold. Hot weather acts as a dampener to lovemaking. Too cold and the sexual heat can get dissipated. The right temperature is when both of you feel comfortable while naked.

Kama Sutra is not limited to the bed alone. In fact, there are many other promising places inside the bedroom itself. You can use props and supports to enhance your sexual pleasure. Many sexual poses and positions require special props.

In case you are planning to use some of the daring and exotic positions described in Kama sutra you can keep the props handy.

A nicely decorated bedroom gives a boost to lovemaking. Don't forget the bedcovers and bed sheets – after all you will ultimately lie down on it during and after a bout of hectic sex. Setting the tone for weekend sex begins with the décor of your home and especially your bedroom. A subtle splash of color enhances sexual pleasure by relaxing you and your partner. Lighting can give a poignancy to love making which you will remember for a very long time. Perfumed candles are available in all supermarkets. You can also order specially perfumed candles online.

Kama Sutra is all for the healthy outdoors. Vatsyayana recommends a tryst in the wild for really rough and uninhibited sex. Nature has everything in abundance – smell, sight, sounds and many sensual delights. The best part is the weather which is unpredictable. You may encounter bright naughty sunshine or a muggy rainy day exuding grey and dark seduction. Making love in the open is an exhilarating experience. You can drown your senses in exotic locales giving a special flavor to your sexual escapades.

You must ensure that you are properly kitted when you dare to move outdoors for lovemaking. Proper groundsheets, bedrolls and tents must be available. You must remain vigilant against animals and insects which may be lounging or crawling around in the natural environment. For some folk, the threats afforded by the open give a new and dangerous dimension to lovemaking, which enhances sexual pleasure.

Food for vigorous sex

The next sense connected with sex is the taste – the fresh taste of your lover's skin, the love fluids which pour out of them and the taste of food before and while having sex. Food and drinks are an integral part of sex. They form a vital part of lovemaking. Vatsyayana, the author of Kama Sutra has emphasized the importance of eating and explained in detail the type of food which must be consumed while making love.

Vatsyayana suggests that lovers must make arrangements for proper food and drinks while planning for extended love making. Obviously the fun would be lost if you were to look for something to bite into in between bouts of passionate sex. There are different kinds of food – some ignite the fire within and provides the required energy to perform. Don't forget that sex demands high amount of energy and vigor from both the partners. In the days of Vatsyayana, there were no canned foodstuff – everything was fresh and natural. It is scientifically proven that fruits and vegetables lose their nutrients when they are preserved. It is therefore recommended to pick up fresh fruit from the market. You can share a few bites of fruit like apple. Feeding each other can be highly erotic and can set the stage for a hectic session of lovemaking. Tropical fruits are known to have aphrodisiac properties. These can enhance sexual performance and take you to an incredible and intense level of pleasure. Honey extracted from wild bees is not only filled with instant energy but can give you a high never before experienced by you. Milk is considered to be an aphrodisiac which must be had during foreplay. Make sure that you don't have lactose intolerance. Fresh milk taken from farm cows fed on natural grass doesn't cause lactose intolerance.

You must remember that too much of anything (other than sex) is bad for health. Don't gorge on food just because you have read that it's good for sex. The stomach must never be full if you really want to enjoy sex. You may feel sleepy and sluggish after a big meal. It is no laughing matter that you fall asleep when your partner is still not satiated. You must avoid red meat and dishes made out of animal flesh. Meat can diminish your interest in sex by reducing the level of sex hormones. In fact, a heavy meal and sex don't go together. There is an added problem with eating a big bad meal – you are liable to belch and even pass air which can upset and offend your partner. Keep your stomach light and your heart heavy is the advice from Kama Sutra. Nibbling on fresh fruits, on the other hand, has many beneficial effects. Studies have shown that the sperm count increases when you consume citric fruit. The modern world is full of couples who wish to have a baby but are unable to do so. Fresh fruits help women to conceive and can be eaten even when you are not in the love making mode.

Consuming wine or other intoxicants was a regular practice during lovemaking during the days of Vatsyayana. Even here, moderation is recommended. You must avoid heavy liquors like whiskey and rum. Couples, especially men get carried away and get drunk before they get into bed. Heavy drinking lowers the libido and you can fail to get an erection when you most need it. You can imagine the frustration which this can lead to. Your partner may be accommodating but a few episodes of flaccid inactivity can drive away women with the best intensions. Therefore it's best to avoid hard liquor.

The flip side of the coin is that mild intoxication can elevate your sex to another level altogether. In the days of Vatsyayana, couples used to enjoy consuming herbs mixed with milk and other liquids which caused intense and strong erections in men and love secretions in women. Eating and smoking drugs enhances sexual pleasure. Make sure that the drugs you propose to have are not banned in your state or country.

Drinking small quantities of wine is good for lovemaking. It gives you a heightened sense of awareness and at the same time you don't lose control of your body. The process of consuming wine should begin before your lovemaking and continue even as you are indulging in the act of sex. You can playfully exchange small sips of wine with your partner. This can be extremely erotic and lead to a great session of continued lovemaking.

Chapter 2 - The heavenly scent of a man/woman

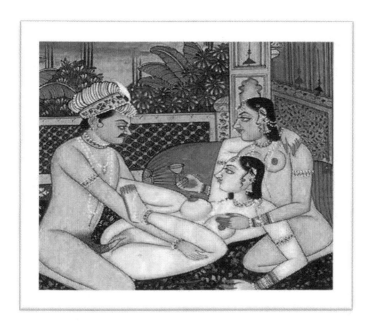

They say that sex is in the air. Animals depend on smell to know if the female is receptive to sex. Remember that only human beings don't have a season for having sex – it's open season for us.

For all other animals, except a handful, there is a specific time for sex. Females are said to be in heat when they are ready for sex. At these times they emit a smell which signals their receptiveness. Though there may not be a specific timetable for us, smell remains an important trigger. Certain smells can easily get us into a frenzy of passion. Our desire to mate becomes intense and the quality of lovemaking also increases manifold when our nose gets a whiff or scent of sex. Of course, humans have lost the sense of natural animal smell , but we have many other ways to seduce ourselves.

Seductive Scents

Kama Sutra suggests many ways to enhance sexual experience by using scents and fragrances. The ritual of sex begins when you attract your partner with perfumes, scents and fragrances. Vatsyayana recommends that both partners indulge in a bath by first applying aromatic and fragrant oil to the body. It is preferable if this is accomplished by the lovers together. Take your time in putting oil on each other's body. You can begin with the tips of your fingers and end with the private parts. This can be deeply sensual and may lead to climax multiple times. Applying oil can be highly erotic if the partners know how to stimulate the sexual organs. In Kama sutra, the vagina is called the Yoni and the penis is referred as Linga. By slightly touching the vaginal walls and stimulating the clitoris, a man can bring a woman to orgasm. Likewise, women can excite the senses of a man by manipulating the Linga. Vatsyayana advises that both partners should try and avoid bringing each other to climax till the very end. This will enhance the pleasure and prolong the sexual ritual.

A ritual bath can also be taken individually. You can pleasure yourself by masturbating and bringing yourself to climax. The skin of a woman becomes tender and supple after orgasm. It also puts you in the right frame of mind.

There is another benefit of applying perfumed oil to the body. It removes foul smell due to sweat and the skin becomes fresh and supple after an oil bath. You can remove the oil by taking a bath or simply let the oil soak into the body. The skin will start glowing and exude an erotic aroma which will be irresistible. Scented soaps can be used to further make your skin smell heavenly.

You can enhance the sense of smell by applying sandalwood paste to your body. Sandalwood is natural and therefore will not damage your skin unlike artificial perfumes which can cause allergy. Cologne is a huge turn on for women. Remember to use a subtle aftershave because strong smell can diminish the effect of other fragrances.

We are fortunate that we have room fresheners which we can spray wantonly. Kama Sutra suggests use of incense sticks and scented candles to provide freshness to your lovemaking chamber. You can sprinkle rose petals on the bed to create a romantic atmosphere.

It is said that smell can bring a dead man to life. This is the power of scents and fragrances. You will remember your lovemaking for a very long time because smells put you in a spell.

Touching and feeling each other

By now you are aware that Kama Sutra goes much beyond sexual positions. Kama sutra is a complete manual for sex which is a must read for all modern lovers who have either forgotten the basics of lovemaking or have never known the true art of sex. According to Vatsyayana, sex is a divine expression which must be experienced in all its nuances and dimensions. Touch is an important and significant part of the sex act. A sensual touch can even lead to orgasm. At the least it is a precursor for explosive sex. Kissing takes a transcendental place in the sexual context. Vatsyayana claims that your lips and mouth are as sensitive as the penis and vagina. Kissing inflames your passion and prepares you for heavenly bliss. Kama Sutra has devoted extensive material to the act of kissing. Lip to lip kiss, caressing of the body parts with kisses, Yoni and Linga kisses have been described in detail. Lovers should give pleasure to each other and build up passion by using their lips to kiss and caress the nape of the neck, breasts, armpit, belly, inner thighs, the sole of the feet an finally the yoni and Linga. The nape of the neck is highly sensitive and responds quickly to caresses. Man should begin by slowly messaging the neck and proceed downwards to the small of the back and then lower still till you feel your partner relaxing and responding to your love caresses. This is the time to go slow and not hurry. Women take more time to get aroused and men should be patient and understanding. Trying to have sex when the woman is not aroused, mentally and physically can be disastrous. Penetration can cause pain and your partner may withdraw completely.

Vatsyayana has described various types of kisses in great detail.

A kiss is the beginning of more fun to come. Lovers begin exploring each other with the 'The Nominal Kiss' in which the lips touch without body contact. The next stage is called the 'The Throbbing Kiss' where any one partner presses and moves the lower lip on the lips of the partner. The transition can take a few moments or minutes depending on the arousal state of each partner. If the partners are involved in light banter, they may indulge in the nominal kiss several times and move away from each other. This situation can be extremely erotic and may even result in transition to a more physical intimacy. 'The Touching Kiss' leads to caresses with hands while the tongue tastes the lips of the partner.

The Straight Kiss, as the name suggests is a kiss when the lips meet directly with a slight movement of the head faces to accommodate the kiss. You may use your hands to touch each other's body gently but without any urgency.

The Bent Kiss is the next stage when the lips contact is intimate and the tongue starts exploring and tasting. Partners hold each other's faces by putting their hands behind the neck. The bodies come closer together and the sense of urgency increases and is felt by both the partners. Holding this position for long may not be feasible or advisable. The Turned Kiss allows one of the partners to hold the chin of the other partner tilted upwards. This position permits the lips to be fully in contact and allows the tongue to probe the partner's mouth and lips.

Kissing is part of foreplay and though it may give intense pleasure, the aim of the union is to achieve a congress of the yoni with the lingam. To achieve this objective you have move on to the pressed kiss. One of the partners presses the lower lip of the other gently with their won lip or finger.

Vatsyayana suggests that lovers should have a tiff or fight during foreplay which will make lovemaking more interesting. Merely having sex and ejaculating is not the goal, nor does it give lasting pleasure. Foreplay adds flavor to lovemaking and extends climax and therefore the pleasure. The Kiss of the Upper Lip is suggested as an occasion to introduce a fight among the lovers. The female partner can wager on who will get hold of the other's upper lip and behave distraught if she loses. She can then move away from her partner who can cajole and coax her to come back in his arms. The Kiss of the Upper Lip involves one partner to kiss the upper lip while the other kisses the lower lip.

Vatsyayana reveals that the upper lip of a female is directly connected to her clitoris through nerve endings. By stimulating her upper lips you can instantly bring her to an aroused state. In The Clasping Kiss one partner holds the lips of other between his or her lips. Wrestling Tongues, means the lips, tongue and mouth come into action. The partners can explore each other's lips, mouth, palate and tongue.

Exploring the Erogenous zones

The kiss is only a precursor to serious sex. Each partner should now arouse the other by kissing the erogenous zones; these are parts of the body which are extremely sensitive to touch. Moving down prom the face, lovers should kiss the nape of the neck and throat. Licking and scratching with the teeth can be erotic and lead the partner to experience extreme pleasure. The female body is dense with sensitive areas. The breasts usually enlarge and the nipples become hard during lovemaking. Kissing these regions can even lead to an orgasm. Women will respond will equal passion to the strokes and caresses of the man. Moving downwards, the inner thigh and back of the calf are extremely erotic and respond to touch. Kissing the stomach is a definite turn on. Sole of the feet can be kissed to elicit an instant response.

Kissing must be accompanied by bites and scratches. Kama Sutra suggests various ways to excite passion through love bites. Scratching is another erotic maneuver which can arouse passion.

The final frontier of kissing is the yoni and the lingam. Kissing and licking the vagina rhythmically with the tongue is known to result in orgasm for women. Kama sutra emphasizes the fact that some women get more pleasure from the tongue of their lover than from insertion of lingam. Some women reach climax only through physical stimulation. The male partner should be experienced to understand the true desire of his partner and respond accordingly.

Women can ignite passion in a man by kissing his lingam. You can either kiss the lingam by holding in your hand or suck on it while it is erect. Sometimes, men may not achieve an erection even after foreplay. Putting the lingam in the mouth and sucking it softly can lead to an erection. Women can use their nails to gently scratch the scrotum while squeezing with the other hand. The skin around the scrotum is highly sensitive and responsive to touch. You can take the lingam in your mouth and suck on it like a mango. You can either gulp the fluid in case your partner has an orgasm or withdraw your mouth to allow the fluid to spill outside. This action can be performed in various positions – while your partner is lying down, standing or crouched.

The male partner should communicate verbally and let the partner know how you feel about the caresses and guide her to maintain the rhythm and pace to achieve orgasm. It is considered appropriate to take permission from the partner before ejaculating in the mouth; otherwise you must pull your lingam out and drain your fluid.

There are different ways described in Kama Sutra for pleasuring the penis. The simplest is to hold the penis in the hand and move it around in your mouth using your lips to put pressure on it rhythmically. Nibbling the penis on the sides accompanied by soft kisses, while holding it from the head, gives intense pleasure. Sucking on the lingam with the mouth holding the head is another way to please the partner. Licking and stroking the lingam alternately gives intense pleasure. Flicking the lingam with the tongue while sucking; wrapping the hand around the penis while sucking and licking; taking the lingam fully in the mouth and sucking, are various ways to pleasure your partner.

Pleasuring the Yoni

While Vatsyayana wrote about woman's sexual desire and anatomy the Kama sutra many thousands of years back, the modern man is still unaware of it. It was known back then that many women find oral sex and stimulation of their sex organ much more exciting than intercourse. Women can be easily aroused and brought to orgasm by using your tongue. The vagina is a highly sensitive organ which has many millions of nerve endings. The clitoris which is inside the vagina can be manipulated with fingers to achieve orgasm. You have to remember that the vagina and clitoris are extremely sensitive and a woman may experience pain if her partner is indiscriminate in exploring them.

The vagina or yoni is considered to be a lotus flower and the clitoris is the bud. Exciting this blossom is both a spiritual and sexual experience. In Hindu religion women are a form of Shakti or primordial energy. They must therefore be revered and respected.

In pleasuring the yoni, men should be extremely careful. Licking and sucking on the vagina can be accompanied by caressing the inner thighs and stomach with your hands. The juices flowing continuously from the vagina are in the form of a clear liquid which can be consumed by the partner. Some women give copious amount of fluids and more so while having orgasm.

The yoni consists of an outer and inner sheath called labia majora and minora respectively. The clitoris is protected by a sheath and lies at the top of the vagina. It's important to know the anatomy of vagina before attempting to pleasure it.

The male partner can simply kiss labia majora or the outer sheath without parting the vagina. If the partner desires, you can part the labia majora and gently lick or stimulate with your fingers. Sometimes women find it painful and may ask you to stop your caresses. You may proceed to spread the vagina by prying open the labia minora if your partner continues to enjoy your action. You should use soft and gentle strokes while licking the yoni. Do not press hard with your fingers unless asked specifically by your partner. The clitoris is the most delicate and sensitive part of the vagina. It gives explosive relief to women and when the clitoris is stroked and licked with the tongue. You can either lick the clitoris along the shaft or directly use your tongue to suck on it. You can feel your partner responding to the strokes by the movement of her thighs. You can increase the speed of your thrusts till she reaches climax.

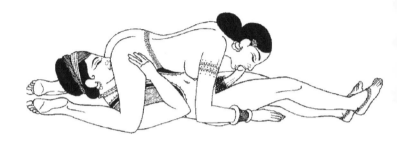

Both the partners, male and female can simultaneously give pleasure to each other with their tongue and fingers. This is called 'Kiss of the crow'. There are many ways for consummating this act. You and your partner can lie down side by side and exchange kisses to the lingam and yoni simultaneously. Other alternatives are man lying on the back with women on top and reverse position.

Prelude to sexual union

Sex according to Kama sutra is multifaceted. There are many dimensions to lovemaking.

Cuddling and embracing each other can also provide sexual bliss. Sometimes couples may simply lie down together after a bout of hectic sex. At these times the body is fully satiated but still craves for physical intimacy. Embraces also serve as a prelude for sex. There are many types of embraces which have been described in Kama sutra.

Embrace of a Twining Creeper

This embrace is in standing position. In the Embrace of a Twining Creeper, lovers embrace each other by entwining their legs and holding each other close with their arms. The female partner, who is usually shorter in height, rubs her thighs and legs by wrapping one leg around the body of her lover. This position may also lead to insertion of the lingam in the yoni of the female. This position cannot be maintained for a long time and is only used as a prelude to other sexual positions which are described later.

Embrace Like Climbing a Tree

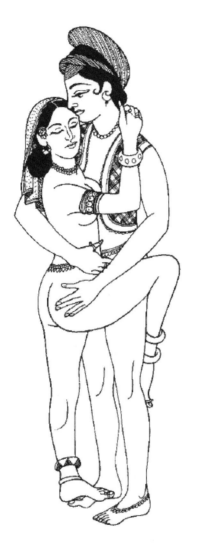

This is another standing embrace. The lovers embrace each other with their arms. The female partner places one of her foot on that of her lover while with the other leg she attempts to raise her legs and rub along his thighs as if climbing a tree. Sexual union can be realized in this position though the lovers have to make certain adjustments to accommodate the lingam and the yoni.

Embrace of Rice and Sesame Seed

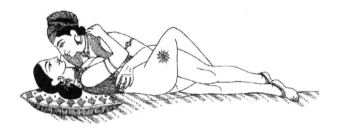

The Embrace of Rice and Sesame Seed is performed in a lying position. The male lover puts one of his legs between the thighs of the female while she wraps herself around his body. The embrace is so tight that it becomes distinguish the partners. This is the reason why it's called rice and sesame seed embrace.

Embrace of Milk and Water

Like there is no difference between milk and water once they are mixed together, the embrace of Milk and Water dissolves the boundary between man and woman. In this embrace, the male partner sits on a bed or in an elevated place while the female places her body across him on the lap. This embrace brings complete fusion of the two bodies and the union can lead to the entry of the lingam into the yoni with total ease.

Embrace of the forehead

This embrace is quite simple to perform. The lovers touch each other's forehead with their fingers and lips. This embrace is passionate and enhances the feeling of love and affection between the partners. The embrace can be either in sitting or standing position.

Embrace of the Thighs

The thighs, especially the inner thighs are highly erogenous. Rubbing of the thighs while in tight embrace can be highly erotic. This embrace usually leads to union of the lingam and the yoni in a beautiful explosion of sex. This embrace can be chosen while sitting, standing or in lying position.

Embrace of the Middle Parts

Sometimes, couples want to avoid penetration but still wish to enjoy the highs of sex. The embrace of the middle parts is highly erotic since the two bodies can rub against each other especially the belly and the thighs, which are erogenous zones. The lingam and the yoni can also seductively rub against each other leading to an explosive climax.

Embrace of the Breasts

In the Embrace of the Breasts the couple can either stand or sit close together with their chests pressed close together.

The blissful union of Lingam and Yoni

Kama Sutra emphasizes that lovemaking is not only about the pleasures of the flesh but also a spiritual union. The focus is not on the climax of sexual union but on the entire process beginning with seduction and foreplay. The problem with our hectic lifestyles is that we miss the substance in our quest for quick results. The focus is on the orgasm and everything else connected with sex is obliterated and ignored. It would have been great if everything had worked out but unfortunately people in this modern world are more sexually frustrated than ever before in the history of mankind.

It is therefore essential to relearn what we have forgotten – to enjoy sex in all its nuances. When two people build up the tempo of their lovemaking the climax is powerful and energizing. It elevates your normal life to a place of supreme ecstasy and bliss. Women reach orgasm much later than men. As a result, they are dissatisfied and frustrated in their sex life. This frustration leads to serious psychological problems which have direct link with society. A thorough understanding of female sexuality, not to mention male sexuality, is critical to the wellbeing of our society. Kama Sutra is great piece of work advising people about the ways of lovemaking and about how to satisfy your partner.

According to Kama Sutra there are three types of Yoni and Lingam. The yoni and lingam have to be paired together according to their size to provide maximum pleasure. However there is no restriction in copulation between other combinations as well.

Depending on the depth of the Yoni there are three types of women - female deer, a mare, or a female elephant. Man is divided into three categories according to the size of his lingam - the hare man, the bull man, and the horse man. There are therefore three equal unions between lovers of similar size and there are six unequal unions, when the sizes do not correspond, or nine combinations.

Compatible unions

The Hare Deer, Bull Mare and Horse Elephant combinations are considered compatible while the Hare Elephant, Bull Deer, Hare Mare, Bull Elephant, Horse Deer and Horse Mare combinations are unequal. Size matters because the woman may not be able to accommodate a much larger lingam if her Yoni is small in size. This can lead to discomfort and woman may not be able to enjoy sex. On the other hand, a small lingam may not derive enough pleasure if inserted in a large yoni. However, other unequal combinations may yield enormous pleasure if the sexual partners are experienced and can stimulate and excite the yoni sufficiently to become enlarged. There are many sexual positions which can benefit couples when the lingam is small in comparison to the size of yoni.

Kama Sutra has divided men into three categories according to the strength of their desire. Men with low desire are supposed to produce little semen and don't enjoy the embraces of a women. They are called men with small passion. Those with a healthy desire are called men of middling passion. Those who exhibit high level of passion are categorized as men with intense passion. Women are also classified in a similar fashion. There is another mode of classification which depends on the time; short-timed, Moderate-timed, and long-timed. The combination and permutation of the two categories gives rise to nine types of unions.

Kama Sutra has described seven types of basic unions in which the partners are lying down. These unions are recommended to couples depending on the type of lingam and yoni. Kama Sutra advices couples to resort to three unions; when the yoni is much smaller than the lingam; deer yoni and stallion lingam. The first three of this exhibit a high level of desire and arousal, since a small yoni must be sufficiently stimulated to ensure perfect union with the lingam: otherwise the female partner may experience pain during intercourse.

The remaining four unions may not be as intense as the earlier unions but they don't lack in intense pleasure and excitement. The reason why they don't involve extensive foreplay is because the yoni is larger than the lingam and does not require lubrication to the same extent. Elephant yoni and a hare lingam is a good example of such union.

The Wide Open Yoni

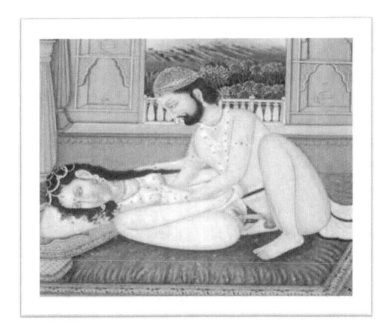

In this posture the female invites the male partner for union with   wide-open yoni. There are three variations to this position. In all these three unions   the woman is in a lying posture – in the bed or on the ground. The male partner is invited to lie alongside her, kneel, or crouch between her legs. The male and female partner faces each other while the man   guides his lingam into her yoni.

Kama Sutra time and again emphasizes the importance of foreplay. Women with small yoni must have a well lubricated yoni for her to enjoy the congress. Foreplay arouses the woman, softens and expands the yoni to enable the fully erect lingam to enter her easily. The male partner should take sufficient care to ensure that any pain or discomfort is avoided.   These three basic positions involve deep penetration bringing the swollen clitoris in blissful contact with the fully aroused lingam. Both the partners thrust their bodies together to achieve orgasm.   The male partner can change pressure and contact of the lingam with the clitoris by changing the angle of penetration.

Widely Open Union

The female partner lies level on her back with her knees up, feet flat, and legs spread wide to allow the man between them. As the man approaches, the woman raises her hips and arches upward to welcome his lingam. The arching upward movement further widens and tilts her yoni to let the male partner penetrate deeply inot the yoni.

The female partner should use the muscles of your thighs to push your pelvis upward. Remember to use the muscles of your thighs to maintain the position without straining the back. Kama Sutra is replete with suggestions regarding the use of props and pillows. These can be used to support the back and other body parts during intense intercourse. Propping a pillow under your pelvis provides a generous opening of the yoni to the rampaging lingam.

This position is highly vulnerable to women. Unnecessary friction between the yoni and the lingam can cause intense discomfort for the female partner. It's the duty of the male partner to ensure that his partner is fully aroused and lubricated before attempting to thrust your lingam in the yoni. The man should gently touch the vagina to feel the wetness. The vagina is also swollen during heightened anticipation. The movement of the female towards the man should indicate that she is ready for intercourse. The woman should be fully aroused to ensure proper penetration.

Yawning Union

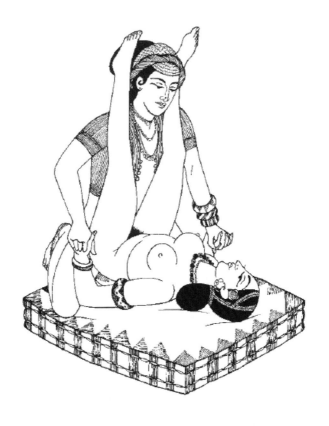

This is another variation of the wide open yoni.
This is a highly erotic and satisfying position
providing extreme pleasure to both the partners.
The female partner lies flat on her back with her
legs up and spread open in a "V" shape. The man
kneels with his thighs spread and guides his
lingam into her yoni. The man's thighs support

the back of the woman's thighs. The man can support himself over the woman with his hands beside her, or the woman can hold his hands to help support him in a more upright position.

It is clear that the clitoris does not get stimulated directly. The woman is restricted in her movement because her thighs are held on the man's thighs. In this position the male partner has a full view of the female body including the vagina. This visual treat increases his desire and the thrusting becomes more intense and pleasurable. The man can change the rhythm, pace and depth of penetration by changing his position marginally. The male partner should look for cues and signs from his female counterpart and respond to her accordingly by changing the pace and depth of penetration. This will give maximum pleasure to her and assist in achieving orgasm.

The female partner must use her hands to change and alter the angle of penetration to derive heightened pleasure. In a variation on this theme, women can   modify the yawning union by putting your legs over your partner's arms and resting them against his shoulders. This pulls your legs against your body while keeping them spread and fairly straight, tilting your yoni upward to increase contact against your clitoris and vulva.

Men should use the thighs to help you thrust so you don't put too much pressure against your partner's thighs with your upper body. In the modified yawning position, slide your knees back so you are pressed tightly against your partner.

Union of Indrani

This position is only for the nimble and flexible bodies. Couples engaging in this union must be healthy and fit.   The woman lies flat on her back and draws her legs against her body, calves touching thighs and knees touching her chest. The man kneels before her and she rests her feet against his sides, spreading her knees apart.

The union of Indrani pulls the muscles of the thighs and hips tight, which both tilts the woman's pelvis upward and opens wide her yoni. The male partner increases the tension of this movement by gently pulling the woman's thighs apart as he enters her. As the woman's yoni is filled with the man's lingam, the woman's buttocks rest against the man's thighs.

The union of Indrani has less clitoral contact than the widely open union. It provides more contact to the perineal area and depending on the angle of penetration, it can also stimulate the woman's G spot.

To assume this position the woman must communicate to her partner her most comfortable angle. You might need to stretch your legs by shifting into a yawning or modified yawning position or relax your back. Also let your partner know if you'd like more clitoral stimulation or extra lubrication.

The male partner must make sure that your partner is fully aroused before you attempt to enter her. Keep your thighs against her bottom to help you control the depth of your thrusts.

Full Body Intimacy

The remaining four basic unions for lying together in lovemaking feature the delight and intimacy of full body contact. The lingam's penetration is shallow, which increases friction. The clasping union is the basis for all four of these unions, which feature rhythmic and gentler movements.

Clasping Union

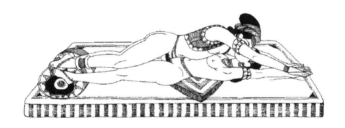

The woman lies sprawled on her back with her legs slightly spread. The man lies on top of her with his legs on the outsides of hers and inserts his lingam into her yoni. The bodies are in full-length contact, which creates a strong feeling of intimacy.

Both of you must kiss and caress your partner's face while looking into each other's eyes to enhance sexual pleasure. The clasping union can also take place when you're lying on your sides facing each other.

Pressing Union

You can start with either variation of the clasping union. When the lingam is firmly in the yoni, the woman presses her thighs together to increase pressure on her partner's lingam.

Twining Union

From the pressing union, the woman places her thigh across the top of her partner's thigh. This draws the man closer to her and pulls his lingam deeper into her yoni.

Union like a Mare

From the twining union, the woman pulls her legs together and contracts the muscles around her yoni to hold the man's lingam tightly inside her.

Compact Unions

Unions in which the woman's legs are drawn up against her body in some fashion are more elaborate unions that open and widen her yoni. Though these unions give the man deep penetration and full contact against the woman's vulva, they severely restrict her ability to move. Many couples find this especially arousing, though it's important for the man to be sure his partner receives the stimulation and pleasure she desires to reach climax.

The female partner in compact unions must stroke and caress your partner's thighs as he thrusts, and push against his body as you are able to increase friction and pressure. Adjust the tilt of your pelvis for more clitoral contact or to control the depth of your partner's thrusts.

Male partners must be careful while assuming this position because your partner's tucked position shortens and opens her yoni and deep thrusting can hurt her. Alter the angle of your thighs to let her adjust the tilt of her pelvis and the depth of your penetration. Stroke and caress your partner's legs and buttocks, and her clitoris for additional stimulation.

Full-Pressed Union

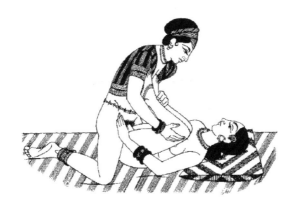

The woman lies on her back, either flat or slightly elevated against a cushion and the man kneels before her. He raises her hips onto his thighs, aligning his lingam with her yoni. She bends her knees and draws her thighs to her chest, and places the soles of her feet against her partner's chest while the male partner enters her.

Half-Pressed Union

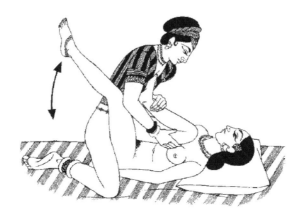

From the full-pressed union, the woman stretches one leg out straight over her partner's thigh. This lets the woman increase the contact between her partner's body and her clitoris, and varies the angle and depth his lingam penetrates. She can move her leg up and down for even more variation in the sensations of their sexual union.

Packed Union

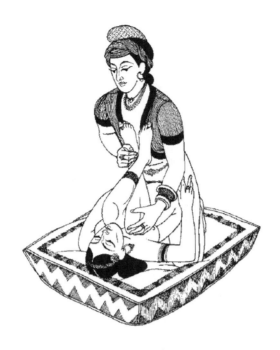

The packed union is similar to the pressed union, except the woman crosses her legs one over the other at the ankles, keeping her thighs tightly together. Lingam and yoni join snugly for intensified friction as the man thrusts.

Unions Imitating Animals

During the time of Kama Sutra, in ancient India, there was a lot of spiritual and religious symbolism attached to imitating the lovemaking positions and actions of animals. Among them, two of the most revered animals were the cow and the elephant.

Union like a Cow

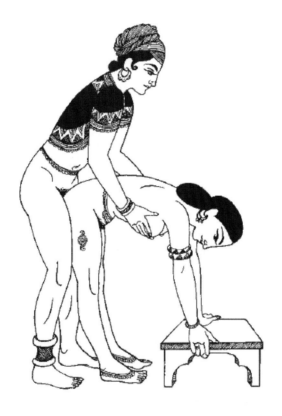

The woman bends over from the waist and places her hands on the floor about shoulder-width apart. Her feet are spread about the same distance apart as her hands, and her knees are straight. The man stands behind her and enters her from the back.

The female partner can place their hands on a low table or bench if the stretch is too much. Tell your partner if you'd like him to stimulate your clitoris to increase your arousal.

The male partner must caress your partner's back, buttocks, and breasts. Use your hand to stimulate her clitoris to give her added pleasure.

Union like an Elephant

The woman lies face down with her hips somewhat flexed to raise her buttocks and her legs slightly spread. The man places himself over her, and draws in the small of his back to insert his lingam into her yoni. Once her yoni encloses his lingam, the woman can press her thighs together to hold it more tightly. The man supports himself with his arms so he can thrust without putting his weight on top of his partner.

The female partner can use a cushion or pillow to elevate your hips for easier penetration. The male partner can draw yourself up somewhat onto your knees and tuck in your pelvis to more easily enter the woman.

Chapter 3 - The Men's Work

The Kama Sutra specifies nine actions that men must perform during sexual union. These movements of the lingam stimulate and arouse the yoni, pleasuring both of them. The man can employ these actions in nearly any sexual union, and should vary them for the greatest enjoyment.

Moving Straight On

Move your lingam straight in and out of your partner's yoni, whether penetration is from the front or the back.

The Churn

Hold your lingam with your hand and move it around inside your partner's yoni, in a churning motion.

The Pierce

With your partner lying flat with her yoni low, guide your lingam into your partner's yoni at such an angle that your thrusts gently strike against her clitoris.

The Rub

Raise your partner's hips so your lingam rubs against the bottom of her vulva and her perineum. You can achieve the angle necessary for this action by pulling her to the edge of the bed and standing as you enter her, or by placing a cushion or pillow beneath her hips to elevate her yoni.

The Press

Press your lingam against the inside of your partner's yoni for as long as it gives   pleasure to both of you.

The Strike

Remove your lingam from your partner's yoni and gently strike, slap, or tap the outside of her yoni with it.

The Boar's Blow

Rub one side of your partner's yoni with your lingam.

The Sporting Sparrow

With your lingam within your partner's yoni, move it up and down faster and faster. This action usually results in climax.

Flexing Your Pelvic Muscle

At the base of your pelvis is a ring of muscle. You're most aware of this ring when it contracts and relaxes to start and stop urination.

Both men and women have this muscle, though it gets far more attention in women. Childbirth can weaken a woman's pelvic muscle, and they are advised to do Kegel exercises to strengthen and tone this important muscle.

Kegel exercises are great for developing control and strength in this muscle during sexual union. The sensations a man feels when a woman contracts her pelvic muscle while his lingam is within her yoni are often intensely arousing , sometimes even more so than thrusting. These exercises are easy to learn, and you can do them just about anywhere and at any time.

Men benefit from toning and strengthening the pelvic muscle, too. Being able to contract and relax this muscle aids a man in controlling ejaculation to enjoy multiple orgasms and prolonged lovemaking.

For men and women, contracting and relaxing the pelvic muscle brings blood and energy to the pelvic area, and a pleasant glow of arousal to rest of the body.

Prolonging Pleasure through Ejaculation Control

Delaying or controlling ejaculation is a sensitive subject for men. Most men are at least a little attached to ejaculating. There is a mistaken belief that sex must always end with a powerful ejaculation. After all, that familiar explosive ejaculation feels good.

But the news is not very good for women. Though men may end their sexual escapade with a spurt of semen, nearly every woman has had the sad experience of being with a man who climaxes too quickly and without warning or apology, leaving the woman wet and miserable. The man usually recedes, becoming disinterested in her still-aroused state and interest in continuing love play. A man who ejaculates and rolls away into his own private reverie or slumber, invites frustration and sexual distress.

Kama Sutra claims that while there is plenty to be said for a man learning to delay his ejaculation to please his woman, there is still more to be found in his learning to delay or put off his ejaculation to experience multiple and full body orgasms. These orgasms occur separate from ejaculation and are at least as pleasurable. The difference is that rather than the intense release that happens with explosion, the orgasm happens independently from ejaculation.

The West and the East view ejaculation differently. In the West, man is virile and strong if he ejaculates multiple times. In the East, the ability to control ejaculation defines a man's physical and spiritual maturity. Withholding ejaculation is believed to be of great physical and emotional benefit to men. A man should monitor his ejaculations with the seasons, his physical and emotional state, and his age. A young man should ejaculate more often than an older man. And those living in a warm climate must ejaculate more frequently than those in temperate or cold climates.

The Pleasures of Delay

The experience commonly known as male orgasm is made up of two stages. First there is an emission as the prostate gland pumps semen into the urethra, followed by the expulsion. The highly pleasurable involuntary contractions of the pelvic muscles pump the semen down the urethra and out the penis. A man can learn to experience and enjoy these stages separately, which enables him to have multiple orgasms.

The benefits of delay ejaculation are many. A woman takes longer to get aroused fully but once aroused, her capacity to enjoy orgasmic pleasure is unlimited. She will appreciate and cherish a man who can delay ejaculation to satisfy her sexual appetite.

The Kama Sutra expresses disdain for a man who does not last long enough to allow a woman full satisfaction in lovemaking.

Such extended sexual loving provides great enjoyment for the man as well as his partner. Controlling ejaculation allows him to fully enjoy the first stage of ejaculation. By interrupting the flow of semen through the urethra, he maintains sexual tension and erection.

Because there is no refractory period following each orgasm, the man can make love until both he and his partner are fully satisfied. This is a practice that requires time to master.

Mastering sexual positions

Kama Sutra suggests some advanced sexual positions which require more flexibility and physical strength than usual. The Kama Sutra presents a number of sexual unions that challenge both the body and the mind. They require practice and concentration— efforts that are well rewarded once you master their physical and emotional levels.

Balance, Strength, and Stamina

Sexual unions that require strength, balance, and stamina also require bodies that are physically capable of performing them. Though some of the sexual unions mentioned here may appear or sound simple, they are difficult to execute. These are unions that, in the time of Vatsyayana, were presented to young lovers as skills to acquire and look forward to over a long period of sexual loving with each other.

Yoga was a daily practice in ancient India, which many of the advanced Kama Sutra unions reflect. These unions require a degree of suppleness and focus that many

Westerners don't typically associate with lovemaking. It's important to know both your own and your partner's capabilities and limitations before experimenting with them.

Requirements for Advanced Sex Positions

Keeping your body in great shape is the first requirement if you plan on going on a single limb. Your body must be toned and flexible. You must develop physical stamina required for prolonged sex. Regular visit to the gym is a must to experience these exotic sex positions. There is a mistaken assumption that only the male partner need be active and agile while the female partner can lie on her back and relax. There couldn't be a more erroneous impression. Both the partners have to be in perfect physical and mental shape to enjoy sex to the fullest - even to enjoy normal sex.

The advanced sexual unions aren't just acrobatic to challenge your physical flexibility and endurance. They are often symbolic—for example, the union of splitting a nail activates the energy of the third eye (the location of the sixth chakra, which governs perception and inner vision). In addition to the physical release that takes place with orgasm, these unions generate a release of emotional and sometimes spiritual energy as well.

Remember that making love shouldn't be a competition or a challenge. It takes a lot of practice to achieve many of these unions, though usually your efforts are well worthwhile. Don't be afraid to laugh and enjoy yourself. It will not work sometimes while at other times it will be a mind blowing experience. Take things as they come. There are many dimensions to sex which you will discover through experimenting with advanced sex positions.

Most of these advanced unions require agility and practice. The Kama Sutra advises that nearly all of these unions take considerable practice to master. Remember, that sex is not only about ejaculation and orgasm, but also to bring each other to deep states of sexual fulfillment— emotionally as well as physically.

Union like a Pair of Tongs

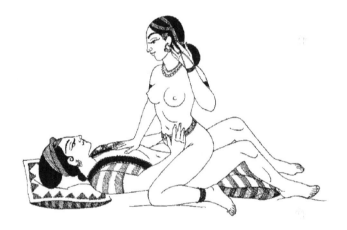

The man lies on his back and the woman sits astride him, facing him. He may leave his legs outstretched or bend his knees somewhat to spread his legs apart. She draws his lingam into her yoni and holds it tightly. She contracts and relaxes her vaginal muscles to press and stroke his lingam. In this way, she stimulates the man and herself.

This union is considered advanced because it takes great control of the vaginal muscles to press the lingam with enough strength and rhythm to create the intense pleasure that will lead to orgasm. The woman may also move her hips slightly to vary the lingam's position within her yoni. Though movements are subtle, this union is one of deep penetration, allowing the woman to direct her own pleasure as well.

Turning Union

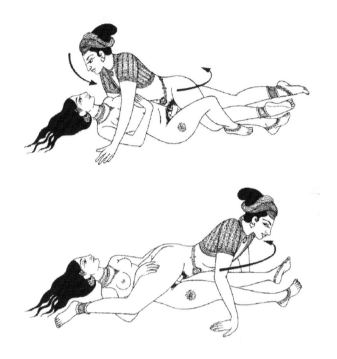

The turning union begins with the woman on her back and the man between her legs. With his lingam in her yoni, he turns his body (taking care not to hit the woman with his feet) until his head is between her feet and his feet on the sides of her shoulders. The objective is to remain within her yoni throughout the movements.

This union gives the woman an unusual and erotic view of her partner's buttocks.

Thrusting is difficult once turned, however. Pleasure is more likely to result from pressing the yoni around the lingam and gentle movements. In the turned stage of this union, the man's lingam is pressing down against the back of the woman's yoni, which may be uncomfortable for her.

The female partner must lie still while the man is turning, to help contain his lingam within your yoni.

Male partner must move slowly and in stages. If you feel yourself slipping out of your partner's yoni, move back to a position in which you can re-enter her. The turning union requires smooth movements and plenty of practice.

Union of Fixing a Nail

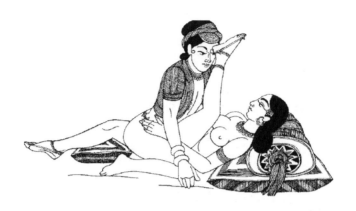

In Union of Fixing a Nail, the woman lies on her back, either flat or against a cushion, with one leg outstretched. She raises the other leg and places her foot against her partner's forehead. Her partner kneels between her thighs, and presses against her raised leg as he thrusts. The angle of the woman's yoni changes with each thrust, as her partner's chest against her thigh moves her up and down. These movements arouse intense sexual passion, though they require practice to perfect.

The union of fixing a nail stimulates the energy of the third eye, which is symbolically located in the center of the forehead. By pressing her foot against her partner's third eye, the woman releases energy that provides clarity, vision, and perception.

Union of Splitting Bamboo

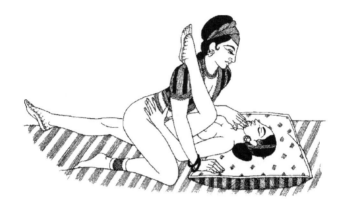

The woman lies on her back, either flat or against a cushion, with one leg outstretched and the other is raised. Her partner kneels before her and rests her raised leg on his shoulder as he penetrates her. She alternates the outstretched and raised legs as her partner's lingam remains within her yoni. Though these movements are intensely arousing, they require concentration and practice. The man can caress the woman's breasts, inner thighs, and clitoris while she exchanges leg positions.

Lotus like Union

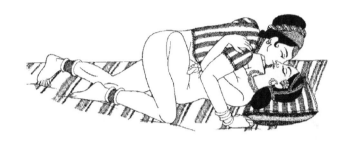

The woman lies on her back and crosses her legs across her midsection, lotus style, with her thighs touching her breasts. This pulls the yoni wide and tilted upward. Her partner kneels over her, supporting himself with his arms, and enters her, with his thighs pressing against hers. Penetration is deep, and there is good contact between the man's body and the woman's G-spot for stimulation during movement.

For women this is a difficult union to achieve or hold for very long, though it can give you intense pleasure. Tell your partner when you've had enough, and slip into a more comfortable union.

Male partners should remember that like other unions that open the yoni wide, the

Lotus like union is pleasurable for the woman only when she is fully aroused. Use your thighs pressing against hers to help you regulate the depth and force of your thrusts.

Union like a Crab

As in the lotus like union, the woman lies on her back with her legs crossed and drawn to her midsection. Her knees point out and stay below her chest, and her feet are tucked under her partner's belly. Her partner kneels over her and thrusts his lingam inside the yoni. Penetration is deep, and the angle of the yoni pleasurably pressures the lingam.

Union like a Spinning Top

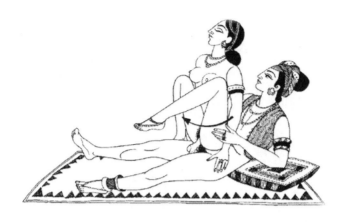

In this position, the man lies on his back with his legs outstretched. His partner straddles him; her feet flat at his sides and her knees up, and take his lingam into her yoni. She slowly and smoothly pivots around until her back is to her partner.

The female partner must move slowly and smoothly to keep your partner's lingam within you and to avoid hurting your partner. Once you've completed your movements and your back is to your partner, lean forward or backward to alter the angle of his penetration.

Male partner must guide and support your partner as she goes through the movements of this union. Caress her back, buttocks, and thighs as she moves up and down on your lingam.

Union like a Swing

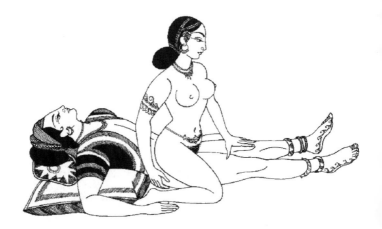

From the union like a spinning top, the man lifts his middle parts after the woman has turned her back fully to him. He then sways from side to side and moves up and down, and his partner rides him like a swing. This requires a strong back and a light woman, and is definitely not something you should try if you have any kind of back problem.

A less straining variation is for the man to lean against a cushion or support himself in a semi-sitting position by leaning against his arms. He can then thrust his pelvis in the described motions without pressuring his back. The woman can lift herself slightly using her thighs and join in her partner's movements.

Supported Union

In this standing union, the woman faces her partner and raises herself to take his lingam into her yoni. The man might need to stand with his legs further apart to lower himself to enter her. The man holds and supports the woman as he thrusts. This union requires good balance. If either partner becomes uncomfortable, just switch to another union.

The female partner must wrap one leg around your partner's thigh for deeper penetration. If you're on your toes with the other leg in order to reach your partner for union, it will be hard to stay in this position for long. Stand on a low stool to equalize your height difference and allow you to stand with your foot flat.

Suspended Union

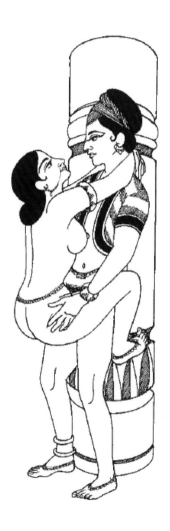

The man stands bracing his back against a wall for support. The woman wraps her legs around the man's waist and her arms around his neck. As his lingam enters her yoni, she hangs suspended from him, pressing her feet against the wall at her partner's back. The man holds the woman's buttocks or thighs and moves her against him. Like the supported union, the suspended union can be intensely exciting though difficult to maintain for long.

Chapter 4 - Post Coital Positions

How often do you linger in the afterglow of lovemaking with your beloved? Or are you busy remembering about grocery list and work of next day? Do you talk to each other and laugh about your love making and the silly floundering that occurred?

When partners continue to touch and delight in each other in after play, the warm glow of their sexual energy continues to nourish the connection they have established through lovemaking as they fall asleep or begin the day's activities. Lovemaking does not have to be an isolated or time-limited event. When you are conscious of how small, shared gestures— lingering together after sex, sharing a passing affectionate pat, kiss, or reminder of the closeness you feel for each other—can extend sexual intimacy, your closeness continues to be a part of the other aspects of your life.

Most couples think that sex is good enough when there has been a reasonable amount of foreplay and both partners achieve orgasm. It is then that men most often retreat to sleep while women often still have more energy to connect emotionally and physically. The discrepancy between the masculine and feminine response to orgasm can be a problem and a source of distrust for couples. Fortunately, partners can find greater intimacy in sex by paying attention to what occurs in orgasm and after.

The Sequence of Sensuous Pleasure

Many people believe that there is still only one kind of orgasm—the clitoral or vaginal for women and the penile orgasm for men. In reality, men and women can experience a number of different kinds of orgasms, some that are limited to the genital area and others that encompass the whole body. Some are powerful throbbing releases that build to a peak and are over, some build to peak after peak of release, and some ride a slow wave across a high plateau and leave the body vibrating for hours.

While both men and women can ejaculate, when a man ejaculates his energy drops off and he requires a period of time to reawaken his erection. This is not the case for a woman. Her appetite is not necessarily diminished by her ejaculation or orgasm. Men can also orgasm without ejaculation, and when he does he can experience a series of multiple orgasms and full body releases that are exquisitely pleasurable. A man who does not experience ejaculation with orgasm usually has continued energy to connect with his partner. Of course, there are exceptions to this.

To understand what happens after climax with ejaculation, it's important to remember what leads up to it. The research of the Western world's best-known sex researchers, physician William Masters and psychologist Virginia Johnson has identified four distinct stages in the cycle of sexual intercourse.

The Four Stages of Loving Making

In the first stage of lovemaking, the stage of enthusiasm or provocation, the body responds to physical stimulation. In both men and women, the heartbeat and rate of breathing both quicken, the skin begins to get warm and flush, and nipples become erect. The man's penis swells into an erection. The woman's vulva and vagina swell, soften, and exude fluid. Her clitoris also swells and hardens. This stage can last up to several hours.

As sexual arousal progresses, the man's testicles enlarge and move tight against his body. The woman's breasts and uterus become enlarged, and her pubic muscle pulses. All sexual sensations intensify as man and woman approach the brink of orgasm. This is the second, or plateau, stage. Lovers can extend this stage by playing the edge or building toward the orgasmic peak, slowing down for a moment or two, and then building again toward the peak a second time, a third time, or as many times as they wish.

The third stage of the sexual cycle is climax, or orgasm. This is an explosive physical release of accumulated sexual energy, marked by intense, rhythmic contractions of the muscles in the pelvic area of both man and woman. Climax is an experience that engulfs the partners, sweeping them into an exquisite pleasure that envelopes them.

People experience the full range from mild to ecstatic states of release and union in orgasm. If you are relaxed at the moment of orgasm and breathing deeply and fully, the contractions that begin in your pelvis can spread throughout your entire body into a full body orgasm.

As orgasm concludes, the changes you experienced in the previous stages begin to reverse. Heart rate and breathing slow. Skin flushing fades. Body parts return to normal size and condition. Man and woman both may feel a sense of euphoria and intimacy.

This is the fourth, or resolution, stage. Orgasm can be elusive for women. Frequently, women learn to have orgasms through masturbation in a particular fashion, and then have difficulty becoming orgasmic during the transition to sexual loving with a partner. In the effort to be orgasmic, many partners become frustrated and try harder and harder to please and be pleased to the point of orgasmic release. Contrary to their efforts, being orgasmic is less a matter of will and more stimulation than it is of relaxing, breathing, focusing on pleasure, and being able to let go of striving for the orgasm. Though orgasm is a physically felt occurrence that can hardly make you shudder or deeply rock a woman to her core; orgasm is an emotional and spiritual occurrence as well. The fear of not having an orgasm due to abusive past experiences, the inability to let go of thinking about future and the reluctance to give up control are ways that a woman prevents herself from an orgasm.

Man's Reaction to Climax

Men who have mastered ejaculation control are able to have several orgasms without ejaculation, prolonging pleasure for themselves and their partners. But once a man ejaculates his ability to have another orgasm ends until his body recycles and he returns to a state of readiness. This refractory period can take 20 minutes to several hours or longer. It is possible for a man to maintain a partial or even full erection for a time following ejaculation, though often the erection fades.

Woman's Reaction to Climax

A woman can immediately have a second as well as subsequent orgasm, and often enjoys the pleasures of doing so. Her body does not require a refractory period, and she can maintain a high level of sexual arousal for as long as her interest and her partner's participation continue. Women who have multiple orgasms may experience them in different ways. One may crash through her body in waves of ecstasy, while another primarily throbs through her pelvis. Not every woman has multiple orgasms, or ejaculates as her orgasms or has them with every sexual union.

Treasure the Experience ... and Each Other

It is easy to see why men tend to consider sexual loving "done" after they ejaculate. A man might feel very relaxed, warm, and "spent," and want to drift pleasantly off to sleep. This is partly physiological—his body won't let him reach a state of full arousal again for a variable period of time. And it's partly emotional or psychological—he feels satisfied, peaceful, and secured.

Most women, on the other hand, are fully capable, when encouraged, to continue lovemaking after one or many orgasms. They desire intimacy and contact after orgasm to complete the experience of sexual loving. Yet many women find it difficult to ask for more attention once their partners have ejaculated.

If both partners approach this difference between men and women with sensitivity and delight, it gives man an opportunity to continue pleasuring the woman or simply be attentive. Sometimes a woman may want to extend the intimacy of sexual union by just lying close and gently sharing strokes and caresses with her partner. Sometimes she may want continued sexual pleasure. Talking about what you are each feeling and desiring is important in creating an outcome in which each feels loved and cared for.

The Kama Sutra repeatedly counsels the man to assure the woman's satisfaction after he has reached his pleasure, warning that a woman left wanting for sexual climax will be frustrated and even angry. There is some physiological basis for this frustration, particularly if the woman doesn't reach orgasm. Both male and female genitalia engorge with blood during sexual arousal. Orgasm releases the muscle tension that makes this possible. When orgasm does not occur, engorgement persists and then slowly dissipates. Either the man or the woman can feel an uncomfortable heaviness and even aching in the pelvic area until the swelling subsides.

Touch

Because a woman's body remains in a heightened state of arousal for longer than a man's, a woman often enjoys continued physical contact and gentle stimulation even if she doesn't desire additional orgasms. A man, too, often finds it enjoyable to stay in touch with his partner's body to extend the shared intimacy between them.

Kiss

Kisses after lovemaking are often tender and gentle. They are kisses to express appreciation and gratitude for the wonderful experience both partners have just shared. They are kisses to express warmth and love for each other. They are kisses that show respect and honor for the relationship and for the union that draws its partners together in body, mind, and spirit. Such soft kisses are calming and soothing.

Stroke

Like kisses after lovemaking, caresses and embraces show affection and tenderness. Lovers lie together and stroke each other's bodies, enjoying the wonder of the ecstasy those bodies have just provided. These touches are gentle and caring, conveying fulfillment and serenity.

Drink

Food and drink can be an erotic and enjoyable part of early love play. You might also be hungry and thirsty now, after extended lovemaking. Feed each other pieces of fruit, cheese, chocolate, or whatever other foods you like. You might enjoy a glass of wine or chilled water. Because you're sexually satisfied, you're more relaxed and at ease. There is no sense of urgency or sexual tension, just the pleasure of sharing.

Bathe

Some partners enjoy bathing or showering together after making love, to refresh and relax. It can be very sensuous to lather, enjoying the heightened sensations that follow orgasm. Bathing together before lovemaking, which tends to be quite erotic and arousing, helps to establish intimacy. Showering together after sexual loving prolongs the familiarity and intimacy of your union. You feel tender and gentle toward one another. If you return to bed and fall asleep, you feel comfortable awakening to another lovemaking session. Others prefer to clean up more privately, retreating for a quick shower and then returning to their partners.

And some people just want to lie together, joined as long as possible, until they fall into the deep and restful sleep of satiated lovers. If they awaken to make love again, they enjoy the feel, tastes, and smells of bodies still warm and moist from the previous session. What you do is more a matter of personal preference than anything else. Some people find the remnants of earlier lovemaking somewhat messy, while others find them arousing. The Kama Sutra counsels couples to discreetly retreat to separate chambers to cleanse themselves, then return to the chamber of their togetherness and enjoy food, drink, and music together.

The key point is to extend your sense of connectedness and intimacy through whatever actions you prefer, rather than separating and falling asleep or leaving. This togetherness is the true culmination of sexual loving.

Cherished Talk

The warmth and closeness that follow lovemaking as you lay together touching and caressing often frees you to talk about the joys of your sexual loving. Many couples feel an especially emotional or spiritual bond to each other at this time, and a desire to extend the pleasure of their lovemaking with tender conversation. They find it easy to suspend many of the inhibitions that might otherwise keep them from sharing so openly and intimately.

Conversation following lovemaking can take just about any course you let it. You can talk about the softness of your partner's skin, the joy you felt when your partner touched you in a certain way, the pleasure it gave you to feel and see your partner in sexual ecstasy. You can talk about the unexpected excitement you felt with a particular movement, or how much you enjoyed trying something different. You can talk about your feelings for each other. Don't talk about the kids, the bills, your job, your parents, and other such potential "hot button" topics. Honor and cherish this time of closeness between you. Real life will intrude soon enough—there's no need to hasten its return.

Laugh Together

Laughing together is a great way to share with each other after the loving. Laughing implies shared fun as well as shared values. It is a way to express your joy and happiness. Lovers who can laugh together can enjoy the humor that naturally arises from human situations. Laughter diffuses discomfort and awkwardness, and can turn a potentially devastating moment into an experience of understanding and pleasure. Sometimes your continued love play will lead to another sexual union as you stroke, kiss, and embrace each other. Subsequent sexual loving can be quite tender, as erotic tension often rebuilds more slowly and luxuriously after it's once been released. Enjoy and explore different sensations as your passion rekindles. This might be a good time to try unions that are more leisurely and relaxed, or perhaps sexual loving that doesn't necessarily lead to union.

Chapter 5 - Couple's/ Partner Yoga

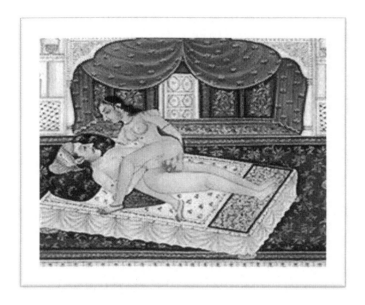

'It takes two to tango' is a popular quote that is true in the case of couple's yoga. There is nothing like couples/partner yoga to hold a mirror up to relationship challenges. In couples yoga both are made to sit back to back and breathe. Moving together both in body and mind is essentially the basic principle of couple's yoga. This helps to erect intimacy, stronger bond and to build trust between both of you. It also enables to make your relationship work at a different level. There is no better foreplay than a session of couple's yoga. Not only does it act like a work out enabling in blood circulation, it also induces sexual desires in both to ultimately end up in bed for a great session of sex.

Immense benefits can be found in the simple, personal practice of couple's yoga. Just becoming aware of self and how you feel can deeply affect the ability to communicate love and your personal needs to your partner. You can wake up to the relationships that are nurturing and begin to recognize those that are zapping you of essential life energy, potentially bringing more love to both. Yoga can create an awareness of space, between each breath, between the incessant thoughts of the mind and between polar opposites of feeling and expression.

How is this possible? Yoga invites us to practice waking up, becoming conscious. It encourages couples to touch each other, awaken their bodies and unite with body, mind and soul.

Stimulates the endocrine system

The practice of yoga asanas, postures or exercises, move the body in such a way as to stimulate the endocrine system. This is the system of glands and hormones that is involved in the way you respond to the world. Balanced hormonal secretion will help to keep the nerve endings coated in the special formulas that ensure that you feel warm and fuzzy as opposed to anxious and distracted.

Breathing exercises also stimulate the elixir of happiness and contentment. By encouraging the movement of the inter costal muscles (the muscles between the ribs) the endocrine system is stimulated. More good happy drugs enter the system like, endorphins and you feel good after a session of couple's yoga.

Here are some poses that can help you to bond well with each other.

Ardha Matyendrasana

Sit back to back and cross your legs with outstretched arms. Place your hand on your partner's thigh and vice versa. Your backs, hips and thighs are in contact with each other. Inhale and exhale at the same time. The rhythmic movement of your body along with breathing helps in making you two gets closer to each other. This is a very intimate moment that can endear both of you to each other.

Badha Konasana

Sit back to back and keep the soles of your feet touch each other. One of you should lean forward while the other bends on you. Your head rests on your partner's back and your chest is expanded. Remember to keep both your backs touching each other.

Anuvittasana

In this asana the man lifts the woman from behind on to his back. The woman's feet are off the ground and she is totally dependent on the man's lift by holding each other's outstretched hands.

Urdhava Dhanurasana

This lift will leave you feeling blissful as the man lies flat on the ground and lifts the woman with his legs on her buttocks. The woman bends her head backwards where the man holds her neck and shoulders with his hands. The woman holds her hands to her ankles and remains in air for a good few seconds. This pose helps both of you to relax into each other and also improve sexual desires.

Aids couple's intimacy

Couple's yoga helps to combine performance and keep fit for yoga and massage. It brings your body, mind and soul together to make it a spiritual experience. The playful act makes couple's feel happy and joyful. It also adds a new depth to your relationship. This is an ideal work out where you can improve your intimacy as well as work out together. In case both of you are busy and don't get enough time together, then a session of partner yoga will definitely add zing to your life. Couple who practice yoga together report that they feel more connected to themselves and each other. If you feel disconnected from your partner for some time, get on the mat together. You might find that you are doing more than yoga together very soon.

The exercises and techniques are designed to strengthen and deepen the practice of sex so that it may be a powerful force for personal and spiritual development. These techniques allow for deep relaxation, a complete combination of the energy of sexual convergence within the intense area of sexuality. You tend to depend and trust your partner more and this deepens and strengthens the bond between both of you. The yogic poses and deep breathing gets you sexually aroused and ready for a romp in bed. The ideal time to perform partner yoga is in the evening before retiring to bed. It'll act like a prelude to sex. Also on a lazy afternoon you can enjoy intimacy and foreplay by performing couple's yoga.

Couple's yoga helps you to connect with your partner without any words. It increases strength, makes you lively and blood flows to all parts of the body.

Yoga in any form helps you to feel refreshed and rejuvenated. Couple's yoga makes two people get closer, reignite their passion and help to enjoy blissful sex together. It also bonds both of you and offers a positive growth to your relationship. Where there is love there is peace and couple's yoga enhances love, lust, peace and compatibility between couples. For men it helps to increase the level of orgasm and staying power inside the woman. It is an ideal cure for erectile dysfunction. Instead of taking medication that can cause side effects simply tango with your partner on the mat and then onto the bed for an uninterrupted session of lasting and satiating sex.

Chapter 6 - Tantra Yoga

John and Jane have been living together as partners for 3 years till John was diagnosed with diabetes. His sugar levels were very high and often vacillated making him feel tired and fatigued. He was on medication for control of sugar. Due to this John had a problem getting erection for enjoying sex. He had low libido and often slept as soon as he hit the sack. Initially Jane was patient but as time passed she was hungry for a romp which she wasn't getting from her partner. John sought advice for his erectile dysfunction from his doctor who advised him to take sex inducing drugs like Viagra. The pill had to be taken an hour before (he planned to have sex) and it gave him erection for a longer while. This made John and Jane happy. Many of their love making episodes lasted for more than the usual time. Though Jane didn't complain about it (rather she was happy) the spontaneous satisfaction was missing for both of them. Their sexual cravings were addressed by Viagra but the emotional satisfaction that is achieved after a sexual intercourse session was missing. That was when John heard about Tantra yoga.

Browsing the internet he came to know that Tantra yoga could help to enjoy lasting pleasure with your partner and also avoid taking medications. The amazing truth about Tantra sex is you can enjoy it with your clothes on like a prelude to love making. Many a days when John was getting only a soft erection Tantra sex excited Jane and kept her satiated though their intercourse that lasted only for a short while. The satisfaction John and Jane got out of Tantra sex was much more than physical pleasure.

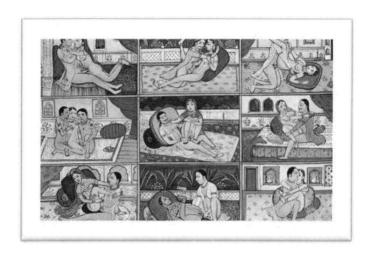

What is Tantra yoga?

According to Hindu scriptures Tantra is a Sanskrit word meaning 'woven together'. Tantra yoga helps couples to enjoy frequent orgasms and multiple sexual climaxes without any disturbance or taking medication. Tantra yoga stimulates the secretion of pineal and pituitary gland thereby offering couples an everlasting body, mind and spirit connection. Tantric sex has a refreshing effect that it helps men and women to enjoy sexual bliss and be rid of several health problems like diabetes, headache, depression, and anxiety, improve weak immune system and also menstrual cramps in women. Tantra believes that the path to enlightenment is only through increased sexual activity. Bhagavan Shree Rajneesh also known as Osho wrote 'Tantra cannot be understood because Tantra is not an intellectual proposition: it is an experience. Unless you are receptive, ready, vulnerable to the experience, it is not going to come to you'. In Tantra the important organ is your mind. The secrets of Tantra are really secretions generated in the cavities (hollows) of the bodily temple.

How to practice Tantra yoga?

Tantra can be practiced both with clothes on and naked as well. The slow removal of clothes as you go along titillates and acts as foreplay. As the sexual energy builds up you can remove each other's clothes one by one. In Tantra yoga you needn't have sex at all. It helps you to relax, enjoy each other's company and aids in building up sexual feelings for each other. Tantric yoga connects couples spiritually and sensually. It enhances soul attraction between couples. Living in the moment with each other without any interruptions will strengthen your relationship. Couples who're aiming to live together for long periods of time should perform Tantra yoga. It aids in keeping them united through body, mind and soul for decades together.

A sexual act can be termed sacred as it unites two people to be together in all aspects of life.

Four Important Poses for Tantra Yoga

Eye contact between couples is very important in Tantra yoga. While making love and during foreplay couples should look at each other continuously. The emotions and feelings you share with each other create a bond and keep you together forever. Tantra sex is erotic, titillating as well as long lasting. The effects are there for people to see. Performing Tantra in the nude is even more beneficial. It makes both of you comfortable with each other's bodies. Here are four Tantra poses that can help you to engage in carnal pleasures and attain multiple orgasms.

Yab Yum

This pose is the most popular pose in Tantric sex. Just as you've the 'yin and yang' in Chinese, Yab Yum means male and female. In this pose the man is seated cross legged and the woman sits on his lap with her legs clasped behind him. Her hands are around his neck and his hands are on her back or buttocks. He pulls her closer to him where his nipples and hers are touching each other. Their faces are close and eyes are open looking into each other. In case you're performing this pose in nude then the man's penis enters the woman's vagina and stays right in. There is no thrusting or thumping happening here. The man takes a deep breath and exhales where in the woman inhales his breath and takes it right into her. When she exhales the man breathes in taking it right into him. In this pose the couples are united in breath, body and mind.

Hot Seat Pose

In this pose the man sits close to the woman from behind. His legs are folded and his buttocks are resting on his ankles. His hands are on the woman's body especially the stomach. The woman is facing away from the man and has her back to him. She is closely seated in the same way with her legs folded in between the man's legs. Her hands are behind on his buttocks for support. In this pose the couple is not looking at each other; instead they are looking in front in the same direction. But the man's penis is inside her from the anal. Both move in tandem up and down or in circular motion exciting each other and building up the tempo. The man's one hand wanders on the woman's body upwards to grasp her breast while the other holds her firmly at the hips. This pose can be tiring; so take breaks when you get tired or too worked up.

Dancer's pose

Dancer's pose can be performed by holding each other for support. The woman's one hand is holding the man's whereas with the other hand she holds her shin or ankle to lift up her leg. In this pose both are standing facing each other. There is eye contact and this pose is performed slowly. Don't be in a hurry to lift your leg high up. Take your time and slowly lift it. Hold your partner for support.

Another way to perform this pose is to kneel down on the floor facing each other. Slowly bend backwards with your head thrown back. Your bodies are touching each other where his penis is rightly touching your vagina. This pose is extremely sensual and erotic. You're only aware of your touching bodies and that connects you to each other. There is no intercourse here. Only touching and titillating each other before the climax where you're sure to enjoy multiple orgasms. This pose can be performed both in the nude as well as with clothes on.

Hand to heart

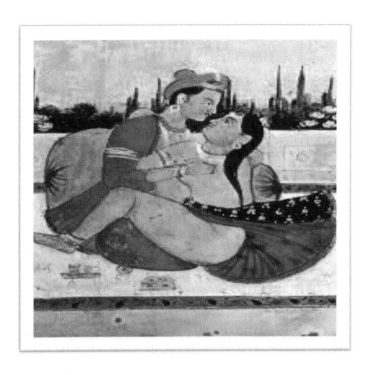

This is a very simple and sweet tantric pose where your hand is on your partner's heart and his is on your heart. You look at each other with a smile on your face. In this pose you can either be standing facing each other or lying down facing each other. This helps you to focus on each other's slow and rhythmic breathing which is an awesome way to converse in silence.

Tantra Massage

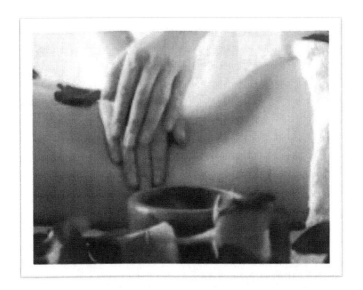

The idea of tantra massage is just to excite each other with tender and sensual touch. Breathe together and look into each other's eyes regularly to form a bond. In tantra massage one partner lies down flat on the ground with the other gently moving finger tips all over the body. This awakens the nerve endings and heightens sexual ardor. Teasing and exciting the other to get an arousal is the basic idea of tantra massage. Tease and gently use your fingertips around genitals and breasts. Don't touch them. Gently tap on the inner side of the thighs and the erogenous zones that heightens pleasure. You can also use tools like oils, creams, fabric or feather. Remember that tantra is only to give pleasure to each other. Sexual intercourse may happen but it is not mandatory. You can just stop with pleasing each other through sensuous, erotic touch and feel satisfied also. The effect of tantra yoga is that you remain in the present totally satisfied and happy. The idea is to unite two people in body, mind and spirit.

Lingam massage

The word Lingam is associated with the Hindu God Shiva. He is worshipped as a Lingam with fervor and dedication. The idea behind lingam worship is that a man's power lies exclusively in his lingam and that power is worshipped as it can cause both pain as well as pleasure. The word lingam is the Hindu word for penis. Worshipping the penis is part of a ritual among Hindus. The meaning of the word Lingam is 'wand of light'.

Gently hold the lingam in your hand and be gentle. Be playful with the surrounding area before you start to massage the lingam. The western world calls it 'hand job'. Do it with utmost care and concentration. Live in the moment and breathe deeply and let out a deep breath. Be slow and take your time. The more time you spend in pleasuring the penis the better your intercourse will be. Once you feel the pressure building in his penis, simply move away from it to the balls or other secret caves of his body. See to it that your partner doesn't ejaculate and climax.

There is a spot between the testicles and anus. That is a soft spot for men. Gently massage that spot with one hand while you hold the penis with the other. Your partner is sure to like it and may have strong emotions come up for you. Be gentle yet stroke him well and sincerely. Once you massage the lingam with passion and dedication you and your partner will reach an absolute level of sheer bliss and ecstasy.

Once your partner is satisfied gently remove your hands and let your man lie in peace and quiet. Allow him to rest for five to ten minutes savoring the pleasure he has gone through.

Effects of Tantra Yoga

Our brain is affected by our endocrinal glands for secretion of HGH, serotonin and testosterone. Studies have shown that health improves when there is sexual stimulation to the brain. It aids in blood circulation, letting out negative energy through breath, strengthening cardio vascular functions and over all keeps a person in good health. Tantra yoga induces sexual urge in couples and encourages people to lead a happy and contented life with improved health and longevity.

Orgasms of 20 minutes or more can alleviate depression making the person cheerful and satisfied. It also improves your immune system and fights aging making you look and feel younger. Oxytocin is produced and there is a decline in adrenaline and cortisol that help in deep relaxation.

If Tantra yoga is performed by a couple then their bond and trust in each other strengthens allowing them to surpass the lower level of consciousness thereby reaching a higher plane of consciousness. Instead of looking at sex as just a pleasurable act Tantra yoga teaches you to perform it as a sacred and spiritual act where both your energies are combined. Also the deep breathing helps to remove negative energy and breathe in positivity.

Tantra yoga and massage helps to reduce stress thereby making you feel emotionally attached to the giver. It helps to refresh, rejuvenate and you feel renewed. You feel the euphoria and excitement once you've enjoyed Tantra yoga.

Conclusion

The ultimate guide to Kama Sutra and Tantra yoga leads to a world of explosive and most exhilarating world of sex. Kama Sutra is not only about sexual positions but provides a holistic and complete view of lovemaking rituals, rites and ceremonies. Using this book you will be able to enhance and experience heightened sex. This is a guide for married couples, partners and lovers. It discusses the entire gamut of sexual experience beginning with foreplay, sexual congress and post-coital rituals.

Kama Sutra encompasses a range of sex related subjects and inspires people to explore and experiment with sex. It actively encourages couples engaging in sex to be free and frank in discussing their innermost desires and physical longings. Sex not only provides physical release but is also a spiritual experience which elevates and enhances lives beyond the normal.

The purpose of this extraordinary book is to provide guidance for couples to experience an exceptional and explosive sexual life. It's time you went beyond the normal and routine lovemaking to a highly enriched and deepened sexual experience.

Other great books by Kathy Lee

Meditation and Mindfulness: How you can learn to Meditate in less than 15 minutes a day like the Ancient Yogis

Made in the USA
Lexington, KY
16 December 2016